42 Ways to Motivate the Sedentary Diabetic to Actually Exercise

Terry R Blankenship

CONTENTS

CHAPTER 1

I REALLY HATE TO EXERCISE:
MY STORY

It was a normal day for me, much like many others. Except that I was to have my long-procrastinated physical from my physician.

No problem … I jumped in the car and quickly navigated the Nashville landscape in the beautiful October sunshine, arriving at her office in about 20 minutes.

Greeting me, we went through the all of the regular tests, exams, etc. She is a very personable doctor and I always enjoyed my visits.

Wrapping up, I thanked her and went on my way.

All was well with the world.

Until she called me a few days later and asked me to come back in for a glucose tolerance test.

"Sure, let's set up an appointment. By the way, why?" I asked.

"Your fasting glucose level came back a bit higher than I would like to see it. This other test can tell us a lot more." she explained.

"Fine, see you then"

Long story short, my glucose tolerance test took about 4 hours with my blood being drawn over and over. I felt like I had given a gallon of blood and was ever so glad to show back up at work that day.

A few days later, the physician called again.

"You have diabetes."

"What? How? Good grief… are you kidding?" I stammered into the phone.

This was the last outcome that I was expecting … the very last outcome.

"Drop by the office to pick up some literature on where to go from here with regards to your diet, medication and exercise" she continued.

To say I was floored is a complete understatement.

I was not only floored, I was totally blindsided with this news. I simply did not see it coming.

I felt it was depressing news. I had zero diabetes in my family history. Zero. And I had always kept my weight fairly steady.

On top of that, I had a natural aversion to candy. Didn't enjoy it so never ate it. How could I possibly be diabetic???

The very next day, I was scheduled to go to Florida for a vacation with some friends. But I knew a couple of things were going to be different.

First, I was going to give up potatoes, white rice, bread, desserts, ice cream and everything else that was high-glycemic index food. And I was going to give it up immediately.

Second, I was going to increase my walking and other exercise dramatically.

All this time, I was testing my blood glucose level with a meter and strips. Usually once a day when I woke up, in order to get a fasting glucose level.

I noticed my dry mouth at night go away almost immediately.

But I was still having some elevated levels.

Fast forward to six months later when I went to Italy and France with some dear friends. I felt that I needed to tell them about my condition since they would be with me so much and observe me passing up pasta, gelato and bread and tons of stuff and would naturally ask why.

They were very understanding.

But that's not the point I am leading up to that I want to highlight.

In Europe, it was very common for us to walk several miles a day. We would walk in many of the medieval towns to see churches, go to restaurants, museums, and a host of other things. It was delightful. And, coincidentally, we were walking nearly 5 to 8 miles a day. It was rigorous and I was exhausted but happy.

(Therein lies a lesson, when you enjoy whatever exercise you are engaged in, you tend to overlook downsides like fatigue, etc)

When we arrived home, I noticed two things immediately.

First, I had lost about 8 pounds even though I'd eaten well.

Second, my blood glucose tests were consistently in the normal range. When I say they were in the normal range, I mean not once were they even remotely in the diabetic zone. Whereas before, I would occasionally get spikes in my morning readings, I never received another spike.

It wasn't long before I went back to the doctor and had an A1 C test and it had dropped from the diabetic zone to the completely normal.

It has stayed this way for the past few years, to the time of this writing.

Do you know how life sometimes serves up lessons to you that, if you're lucky, you will immediately recognize and operationalize the truth that is being given to you?

Well that is what happened to me after my Europe trip. It hit me that my increased level of exercise was the final piece of the puzzle that needed to be put into place.

For reasons that we will discuss later, exercise at a higher level activated a response in my body that was very favorable to my diabetes and its elimination. This revelation came crashing in on me like a tsunami. It was very apparent to me that by simply increasing my exercise, my diabetes virtually was eliminated. It was definitely an ah ha moment for me...

I felt I had discovered the pearl of great price in diabetes management, as it were.

Keep in mind that I am one who hates exercise. I seriously hate exercise. I cannot stress enough how I loathe exercise. Walking on a treadmill to me is about as much fun as having a colonoscopy without anesthesia.

Even though I hate exercise with such an extreme passion, I was forced to admit that it was extraordinarily valuable to me in the management of my diabetes. And because it is, I had to do it no matter what.

So I had to find ways to do this that did not cause me to lose my mind through boredom or whatever. It was simply mandatory that I figure out how to exercise every single day.

I do not completely know how God has made me however I do know that exercise does not come easily or naturally to me.

But I had to find ways to continue the high-level of exercise that I experienced in Europe.

I had to find ways to do this in order to manage my diabetes well.

And that is why I am writing this book. Because I am essentially sedentary and activity challenged. I would rather read a book than ride a bike. I would rather watch a movie then walk a mile. This is who I am and this is how I was composed as human being yet I had to find ways to change.

This book will apply to either you or someone that you care for. Perhaps you are a diabetic yet you know deep in your heart that you need to find ways to exercise and if you are exactly like me, even thinking about exercise is abhorrent. Or maybe the thought of exercise does not repulse you, yet you simply are not able to overcome the inertia and get out the door and do something.

So I thought if I could come up with some ways to launch your rocket out the front door, it would be a good thing. I want to launch your rocket out your front door. If after reading this book, your rocket has not ignited yet, I will have failed in my mission.

If, after reading this book, you are still overcome with inertia, I would invite you to e-mail me at terry.blankenship@ outlook.com for further motivation because indeed, you have a supersized challenge on your hands.

I shouldn't have to say this but I will anyway... you need to check with your doctor to make sure that any exercise that you begin is compatible with your condition. For instance, if you have painful diabetic neuropathy in your feet, don't try to take up running unless you tell your doctor first and listen very carefully to what he says back to you. Promise?

Also, I am a type 2 diabetic. Type 1 diabetics can benefit from exercise immensely but have a differing underlying condition than type 2.

Okay, let's take a look at some ways to get you out of your easy chair and on your way to a better life!

CHAPTER 2

WALK BY YOURSELF

Seriously, this is the very easiest way to start. As a matter of fact, walking was what convinced me of the extreme value of exercise on my diabetes.

This is how easy it is to start... get out of your chair, walk to the front door, open the front door, pass through your front door, find a sidewalk or street that is safe to walk on, start walking, finish walking, go back to your front door, open your front door, pass through your front door, close your front door, now resume your seated position.

Walk for five minutes initially.

Make your walk enjoyable. Look around. Greet people. Look at the birds. Whatever you have to do to make your walk enjoyable, do it.

Studies show that even five minutes walking every day will confer healthy benefits on you. Obviously we want to get beyond the five minutes but we are working at ground level here and if I can get you out the door and walking for five minutes, then this is a victory.

Mark Twain once said, "The secret of success is getting started."

Thomas Jefferson said, "Walking is the best possible exercise. Habituate yourself to walk very far."

I love both of these quotes because taking the first step is the toughest step and once you do it, making a habit of it is truly a super thing to do.

See the appendix at the back of the book for the science backing the effects of exercise on diabetes.

CHAPTER 3

WALK WITH A BUDDY

The magic of walking is that it confers so many benefits to you that it is difficult to list. Suffice it to say that walking is extremely beneficial for managing your diabetes.

Just as my first tip was to walk by yourself, My second tip is to find a buddy to walk with. We are social animals and there is something magic about harnessing your efforts to that of another person. It might be your spouse, a friend or neighbor, a child, or whomever. I really don't care where the buddy comes from but the buddy can provide sorely needed motivation to get you out the front door.

And after all, this book is about motivating you to overcome your inertia.

Here's a challenge:

List 3 possible walk buddies below and invite the first one on the list to do a 5 minute walk with you. If they cannot, move to #2. And # 3. it may be that the buddy can only walk on Monday and Wednesday while another one can only walk on the weekends and you may have to mix and match. But it doesn't matter, does it? Our purposes will be achieved regardless how the puzzle is put together.

Possible walking buddies

1 _____

2 _____

3 _____

CHAPTER 4

WALKING TOURS

We were in Chicago recently for a convention and the weather was simply amazing. You know the types of days, I'm sure ... temp in the low 70s, slight breeze, just perfection. I've always been a huge Frank Lloyd Wright fan, loving his architecture, when I discovered there was a walking tour of some of his homes in Oak Park, a suburb of Chicago. We had a ball, walking and enjoying the incredible architecture that spread before us. (The walking tour map cost $5.95, what a bargain!)

An incredible way to increase your walking is to participate in a walking tour. This does not have to be exotic or expensive in order to be effective. There probably are walking tours in your home city and if not, there are walking tours in a city near you.

The beauty of a walking tour is that they are often highly interesting and you also get the benefit of exercise. During my Europe trip, I did not notice all of my walking because we had so many interesting places to visit and things to see. A walking tour is a great way to ease you into walking if you're just too stubborn to do it any other way... And some of us are, aren't we?:-)

For a great list of walking tours by city, go to tripadvisor. com and you will find a wealth of information.

CHAPTER 5

GET BACK ON YOUR BICYCLE

You know, the one that's parked in the garage that you haven't been on in ages. Did you know that your bike could be possibly one of your greatest fitness tools?

The great thing about bicycling is that it is extremely low impact and also delivers very high aerobic benefit.

I must warn you, before you get back on that old bicycle, make sure it actually works in that your tires are properly inflated, your brakes work, and your chain is lubricated. There is nothing beneficial about getting hurt while trying to get in shape, right?

Bicycling is one of the most helpful things that I do, in addition to walking. I have an 11 mile route through a park in Nashville that is composed of hills that I do regularly. It is extremely low impact however it is strenuous as far as aerobic exertion goes. I know that at the end, the exercise benefit that is conferred upon me is enormous.

By the way, I do not stop at the 11 mile loop… I have taken 20, 30 and 50 mile bike rides. However we are talking about you and getting you in motion so the best way to do this if you're interested in bicycling, is to make sure your bike works (or buy a new one), jump on it and ride up and down the street in order to acclimate yourself.

Most cities have bike paths or online suggested biking trails. Nashville, for example, has an incredible series of greenways on which one can bike.

"But I'm too old to ride a bike", you protest.

Hogwash, I say. If I had a nickel for every 70 and 80-year-old that I have seen on a bicycle, I would own a small fleet of yachts.

You need to read the fabulous book, *Bike for Life: How to ride to 100.*

CHAPTER 6

BIKE WITH A BUDDY

Again, this book is about motivating you to overcome your own personal inertia and resistance to exercise. I know I know I know, you hate to exercise and as you know, I do too.

But we have to get out the front door.

All of the wonderful benefits of bicycling will be conferred on you only if you actually do it. A great way that I have found to make this enjoyable is to get a buddy to do it with me. You will enjoy the other person's company and you will be at least 20 times more likely to bicycle than if you're left to your own wiles to do it by yourself.

I have a friend who loves to bike and is usually up for it whenever I give him a call. He is my biking buddy and I look forward to biking with him.

I know that at the end of any bicycling, my type 2 diabetes is being managed in a very therapeutic way.

CHAPTER 7

BIKE WITH A GROUP

Most cities have at least one bicycle shop. Larger cities have several. Nashville for example has over 20. And in each bicycle shop, there are usually circulars that advertise group bicycle rides at different fitness levels.

Locate a bicycle shop near you, go there, inquire as to any group rides that might be available at your fitness level (which is beginner) and if there is one that fits you, take note of the day, time and place and show up with your bicycle. They are loads of fun and will not stress you out in the least.

"But I'm too old to do anything like that" you protest.

You already know what my response to this is.

CHAPTER 8

BIKING TOURS

As with walking tours, there are an abundance of biking tours available throughout most cities in the United States.

If you are having trouble getting started doing anything and enjoy the idea of bicycling, this could be a great way to get you off of your couch and motivate you to stick your toe in the water.

The beauty of a biking tour is that it is so enjoyable, you are being socialized with your peers, and you're getting exercise while all of this happens.

During my Europe trip, I noticed so many group bike tours that I was astonished. Many of these folks came from the United States but many came them all over the world. They were having fun, being socialized, and getting exercise all at the same time.

The good news is you don't have to go to Europe to do this (although if you want to, it's a great thing to do!). There are biking tours in virtually every city in the United States.

Remember, I am trying to light a fire under you and this is one more match that I will strike if it gets you moving!

CHAPTER 9

JOIN A SPIN CLASS

Spinning is basically riding a stationary bicycle. A spin class however, takes a rather boring activity and throws fun and sparkle all over it.

Most YMCAs and other fitness centers, have spin classes. Typically these are 20 or more stationary bicycles in a large room, that are utilized for a group activity lasting from 45 minutes to an hour with an instructor leading it to the melodies of great music.

To say that this is fun is a huge understatement. It is incredibly fun!

And it is low impact and high aerobic. Almost a perfect exercise. And since you are spinning with other people, the added benefit of socialization is baked right into this.

So many people in spin classes make friends with each other and this serves to motivate each other to higher fitness goals.

It is not uncommon to see people of all ages in spin classes. I'm talking about from teenagers to young adults to middle-age to senior citizens. The spin class I go to has a fellow by the name of Ollie who sits in the corner and participates enthusiastically. He has been doing this for at least 10 to 15 years. Ollie is 80 years old. He is in great shape. I do not know if he has diabetes or not but that is beside the point, isn't it? He may not have diabetes because his fitness level may have been forestalled. Or if he does, he is helping manage it well.

I challenge you to go to your local YMCA or fitness center and see if there is a spin class. The instructors are extremely sympathetic to beginners and you can get in a spin class and going slowly for the entire period of time and no one will say a word because they understand you're starting out. Who could ask for more than that?

CHAPTER 10

DO YOGA

Okay, this may not be the most aerobic of exercises however yoga is a fantastic way to center yourself and open up peaceful avenues within your own spirit. It will also start your body being acclimated to movement and that in itself will confer a host of health benefits upon you.

Most YMCAs and fitness centers have yoga classes. My wife is a very devoted yoga practitioner and will attest to the fact that it helps her mental clarity, her sense of well-being, her sense of peace as well as her sense of fitness.

The great thing about yoga is that it can lay a foundation for you to move into other areas of activity. It is a gateway, in a sense.

What are the benefits for a diabetic? Many studies show that being able to elicit relaxation response from your body has a beneficial effect on your blood sugar.

The Center for Yoga and Health writes on their website: "While the science of yoga for diabetes is still young, there are now several studies, published in peer-reviewed medical journals that suggest clear improvements for people with diabetes. Findings from these small but high-quality, randomized, controlled clinical trials have shown significant improvements in blood sugar levels as well as improvements in lipid profiles, blood pressure, body weight, and oxidative stress (a metabolic imbalance) in participants who practice yoga and meditation on a regular basis."

CHAPTER 11

RUNNING - ARE YOU KIDDING ME?

Okay, if you're truly sedentary then this will need to come after you begin walking or biking. But do not discount this. We are a nation of folks who run from age 10 to age 100.

Oh yes, diabetic folks run also. And the benefits are similar to walking except up a notch.

I will not go into the details of a complete running program but remember this book is about giving you a number of ways to ease into exercise. Diabetic or not, running is fun for a lot of people.

And when I say running, I am talking about everything from jogging which I would define as about 3 1/2 miles an hour all the way to fast running which by my definition is over 6 miles an hour.

There is something about running that is hugely satisfying. I am a runner and as such, run often. I am not a fast runner and probably more of a fast jogger or a slow runner, if we had to categorize. But it doesn't matter, does it? What matters is that I'm out there doing it and you can be out there and do it also.

Your blood sugar control will be wonderfully helped.

Of course you would start off slowly, perhaps running only 100 yards and then increasing it a bit more every week, all the while listening to your body. Oh by the way, make sure you have good running shoes before you do this as you could really hurt yourself with some poor shoes.

There is a really good website that has a program to turn a couch potato into a potato who will eventually jog a 5k route. www.c25k.com

It is slow and gradual and a wonderful way to start out if this interests you in the least.

CHAPTER 12

RUNNING WITH A BUDDY

Much like walking, running with a buddy is a tremendous way to start and maintain an effective running program.

It's that old thing called accountability. Accountability has magic... accountability has motivation built into it... accountability propels you to do things that you would not otherwise do, like exercise.

CHAPTER 13

RUNNING IN A GROUP

Running in a group brings a special type of motivation that is hard to find anywhere else. Obviously, the magic here is exactly the same as walking in a group or doing any activity. We are social animals, designed by God to enjoy and interact with each other. Harnessing this truth about ourselves can bring massive motivation to even the most sedentary of those around us.

Mary had always loved the thought of running but had found herself a couch potato, moving very little during the day, only reading books and watching TV. However, she had developed Type 2 diabetes in the past few years.

Determined to somehow break out of the sedentary cycle, she overheard someone at church speaking of a group of folks about her age who jogged three times a week, at their local Y. Intrigued, she dug out some old running shoes she had and timidly showed up at one of their meetings. Long story short, the group jogged pretty slowly and she fit right in. She loved it.

Because she enjoyed the diverse personalities in the group, she went back a second time ... then a third ... and soon it became a habit. Her symptoms improved and her A1C score fell to the normal range.

Most larger cities have one or more running clubs. For instance, Nashville Tennessee has the Nashville Striders. The Nashville Striders has several group runs every week. A private athletic store in Nashville, Fleet Feet Sports, has several running groups every week also. The point is, it should not be hard to find a group to run with and trust me, they go all the way from the slow joggers to the fast runners.

Again, the most difficult part here is going to be making initial inquiries and contact. Once that is done, you will be on your way!

Remember, all exercise benefits your diabetes as well as a host of other things.

I'm trying to simply get you out the front door.

CHAPTER 14

BOOT CAMP ... SERIOUSLY?

Just about every YMCA or fitness center offer some type of boot camp in order to help people like you and me... in other words, these boot camps are designed to get the sedentary person jumpstarted into a more active routine.

What can I say... this works for many people!

Tom was a person who was a retired executive with type II diabetes. He has never been active, always allowing his career to crowd virtually everything else out including self-care. So if you were to look for the word sedentary in the dictionary, Tom's picture would appear.

He heard about a boot camp at his local fitness center. At the urging of his spouse, he took a deep breath and called the center inquiring about the boot camp. The person on the other end must've been a great salesman because Tom found himself at day one of boot camp about a week later.

Long story short, he loved it.

The instructor tailored every activity for the fitness level of each participant. This began Tom on the pattern of activity that he continues to this day. He just had to give it a try.

He found his insulin resistance going down as he exercised. He was able to cut his medication a bit and found several symptoms of his diabetes going away.

Did I mention that he lost weight also? The hardest step regarding a boot camp is the first one... simply inquiring about its schedule.

But a boot camp can seriously be an inertia killer and that is what this book is all about.

CHAPTER 15

JUMP IN THE POOL

Swimming just might be the very best exercise there is. It is low impact and high aerobic. And you are as likely to find swimmers over age 80 as you are under the age of 30 in any fitness center or YMCA pool.

The downside of swimming obviously is that you need a pool. With walking, you just put your shoes on and walk out the front door. With swimming, you need a pool.

Not a problem, virtually every fitness center or YMCA has one and they usually are parts of the fitness center that open before any other part, often before five in the morning.

If this appeals to you, take the first step and find a pool. Overcome the inertia and locate a facility that will accommodate you. Trust me, it's not hard.

There's even a competitive swimming program called Masters swimming for those adults who would like to compete in swim tournaments. I have gone to a few of these and there is nothing more heartwarming than seeing a few 70-year-olds battling it out in the backstroke.

When they get out of the pool, they look far better than most of their peers and if they are diabetic, they have added satisfaction of knowing that they are doing something wonderful for their condition.

CHAPTER 16

BOOKS

I have always found books to be very motivational in helping me do anything. A great way to help you overcome your resistance to exercise and activity is to always keep a book on hand that is motivational regarding exercise.

I don't know what it is but whenever I have a motivational book that I am working through on some aspect of my life, be it exercise, eating, money, etc., I tend to do far better. In other words, it helps me to focus tremendously when a good book is constantly feeding me motivation.

Remember, this book is all about getting you out the front door and into an activity in order to help manage your diabetes. Whatever it takes, we're going to do it, right?

Here are some good books that have been very impactful to my life:

Younger Next Year

Sharp

Brain rules

Bike for life

Hello New Me

1% Fitness

The RBG Workout

Speaking of *Younger Next Year*, this is a wonderful book by Chris Crowley. One day I picked this book up and began reading it. I could not put it down. He writes in such a clever and witty way that it drew me in and even though I hate to exercise, this book alone got me started. Let me say that one more time... This book alone got me started.

This book is chock full of motivational wisdom, hilarious stories, and text that is designed to rocket you out your front door.

This book so moved me that I recommend that it to quite a few of my friends, and they all loved it. As a matter of fact, even today, after several years, we will all check up on each other and say "have you had a younger next year week?"

Get and read this book. Not optional. Available from Amazon and other great booksellers.

CHAPTER 17

FOLLOW AN EXERCISE BLOG

In much the same way as a motivational book on exercise helps us get out the front door, following a blog does the same thing only the content tends to be much fresher.

Getting a blog delivered daily to you or accessing the blog daily is a terrific way to keep motivation high. If you're like me, motivation to exercise is not something you're born with. It is something you have to work at very strenuously.

Here are a few blogs that I find to be fabulous as far as motivating a person to exercise; they will get you out the front door and keep you out the front door:

Tony Gentilcore

YogaDork

Blogilates

ACE Fitness

The Fitnessista

"Off-the-couch-today.com (this is my blog, please follow and share)"

CHAPTER 18

FOLLOW AN EXERCISE PODCAST

A podcast is a great way to get an audio boost to keep one fired up about exercise. Regardless of the exercise that works for you, you're going to need motivation to keep at it. I don't care if it's walking, running, swimming, biking, etc. etc., it all takes motivation.

The great thing about the podcast is that you can put the podcast on your phone, and walk and get a daily jolt of motivation before your fires go out. Remember, it is the fires of motivation burning low that we are targeting in this book. We are trying to get you out the front door and back into exercise.

There have been many days that I have felt like a slug and was about as inclined to exercise as I was inclined to go jump off a cliff. I needed some external motivation and I needed it fast or else the day was going to be gone with me setting new records for being sedentary. I would get one of my favorite activity podcasts out and listen to a new episode and it would work wonders for me.

Here are some pretty good fitness podcasts:

Motivation to move

Fit Girl

Dr. Fitness and the Fat Guy

The Jillian Michaels Show on Podcasts

NPR | Exercise : Learn To Love (Or At Least Like) It

Quick and Dirty Tips | Exercise Podcast

Shrugged Collective Podcast

CHAPTER 19

WRITE ABOUT IT

Believe it or not, studies have shown that if you keep an exercise journal daily, this by itself will give you motivation to get out the front door. Studies have also shown that as you record your obstacles, challenges, dead zones as well as your successes, you will exercise at a more consistent pace than the person who does not do this.

As I have alluded to before, the toughest step to take in any exercise program is the first step. Any advantage that we can get on our side to get us exercising and keep us exercising, we should take and embrace it enthusiastically.

So go buy a small notebook that you can write in and start today. If you have an iPhone, droid etc that you can keep a journal on, by all means do that! The manner of journaling does not matter... that you do it is the only thing that does matter.

CHAPTER 20

SENIOR OLYMPICS

There really is nothing better than having a structured event or series of events to pump motivation into a person.

If you are 50 or older, the Senior Olympics might just fit your bill. This is absurd, you might say. But wait before you dismiss this idea out of hand. Every year over 50,000 Americans compete in the Senior Olympics. It is not some freakish, odd idea. It exists in every state and draws from all walks of life.

And all of these people have gotten out of the front door. Obviously the goal here is not so much to the win a gold medal as it is to get a person into activity and exercise. Diabetes can throw a person into depression quite easily and that means no activity so something like the Senior Olympics can really help repel the tide of inactivity in a person's life.

Consider this blurb from The Baltimore Sun in 2006:

"Judith Stillman isn't the least bit surprised when she comes home from work and finds a note from her husband saying he's "gone for the day." She knows exactly what he's up to - one of his twin passions of volleyball and softball - and she approves completely. Richard Stillman, 73, is a lifelong athlete who is happy to be "involved in some form of sports just about every day of the week." "You don't have time to think about slowing down when you keep busy," said Stillman, who plays with two replaced knees."

Here is their website - NSGA.COM - visit it and deal a blow to your inertia.

CHAPTER 21

GET A TRAINER / COACH

Studies show that accountability is key when breaking out of an old pattern and embracing a new pattern. This is why so many people find that it is important and helpful to get a trainer for two or three sessions at your local health club or YMCA.

The trainer will show you the correct way to do your exercises, whether they be aerobic or strength. Once you get the hang of it, you are on your own. Many find it helpful after that to, every three months or so, sign back up for another session to make sure they are on track.

This is an option that does not cost much money and can absolutely change your life. It is not for everybody but if you have a really really really bad case of being stuck in the mud and just can't get out the front door, I recommend this.

CHAPTER 22

5K

Walking a 5K is a blast. A 5K is five kilometers which is about 3 miles. Most people can do this distance.

What makes a public 5K so motivating is that they often are organized around charitable events. So in addition to helping a good cause, a person gets exercise.

Often we need to do something like this periodically to blast us out of our comfort zone. There is nothing like an event to transcend our everyday circumstances and get actually moving forward. Especially if we do it with someone or a group of folks.

Obviously this is not restricted to just 5K walks and or 10k walks. But any type of structured event of this type is very helpful.

CHAPTER 23

MOTIVATIONAL QUOTES

There is an old saying that when you go to church, mosque or synagogue, you never really learn anything new, but you are reminded of important things that you already know. And that is extremely critical.

I don't know about you but constant reminders in my life help keep me on track. It is a best practice to surround yourself with snippets of quotations and reminders that will keep you energized and moving in the right direction.

Place motivational quotes all around your house and office. Put them where you can see them or else they will not make a difference.

Even simple quotes like "daily exercise will help my diabetes" are extremely powerful to getting you into a pattern.

This is not expensive... you can get index cards and post it notes and write the quotes on them with a sharpie and then place them wherever you will see them. Trust me, it makes a big difference.

I mean quotes on your bathroom mirror, in your car, on your refrigerator, on your bedroom door, on your iPhone, droid, quotes any and everywhere are a super idea.

Here are a few quotes you can start with:

Exercising daily helps manage my diabetes.

Even a 5 minute walk daily can improve my diabetes.

Move ... move ... move!

Sitting on the couch does not help my diabetes.

Have you exercised today?

Get up and out the front door NOW!

As my exercise increases, my blood sugar decreases.

A couch is NOT a part of my anatomy!

CHAPTER 24

REUNIONS

For the older crowd reading this, as we start hitting our 25th high school or college reunions, you better believe we don't look a whole lot like that skinny kid that graduated way back when.

This book is all about motivating you to exercise in order to manage your diabetes better. It is very motivational to want to look your best at these reunions. Use that desire to place your best foot forward in order to get you into a regular exercise routine.

I know, I know. You hate to exercise... so do I. Join the club. But we must if we want to manage our diabetes well.

So hook that desire to not look like Jabba the Hut at your upcoming high school or college reunion in order to get you out the front door and into a pattern of exercise.

CHAPTER 25

REMIND YOURSELF VIA SMART PHONE

This follows as a first cousin of the reminder category. Only we're using smartphone reminders to do this. On most of today's smartphones, you can set recurring reminders that will pop up at the assigned time daily.

Usually these will make a noise so that it gets your attention and you will look at the smartphone and boom, there will be your reminder.

Use the reminders that I have shared earlier as starters to help you stay focused on getting out the front door and getting into exercise.

Trust me, every little bit helps ...

CHAPTER 26

SCALES

Okay, this might be a controversial one but I want to help you shape your opinions of scales on which you weigh.

Although I know this is not the case with you, pretend that you are a little overweight. We both know that extra weight exacerbates your diabetic condition, don't we?

I have found it very motivating to keep a daily weight journal and see the correlation between the amount I exercise and how much I weigh. This is not meant to be a scientific exercise but there is a truth here. That truth is: what we measure tends to improve. Ponder that last sentence.

Seeing the scales go the wrong way with your weight is an enormous motivation to getting out the front door. Seeing the scales go the wrong way with your weight is an enormous motivation to stop that trend.

More than once, I have become aware that I might be gaining a few only to step on the scales in the morning (BEFORE coffee!) to take a check point. When the scales sing a sad song to me, instinctively I find myself motivated to move more, to exercise more.

Weighing daily, weekly or periodically can tend to improve your weight and can also provide fresh motivation to get out the front door and break your sedentary cycle. Ask me how I know.

CHAPTER 27

GRANDKIDS

Let's face it, for many of us who have grandchildren, they're very motivating. We want to be examples. We want to be our best. We want to control our diabetes so that our quality-of-life goes up which will obviously impact our grandchildren in a positive way.

Visualize your grandchildren when they are grown and further visualize a conversation you might have with them about the importance of staying physically fit when one has diabetes. It is all about example.

Does that motivate you? It does me.

If this is motivational to you, do it. Have that imaginary conversation and think about how you can be an example to your grandkids.

CHAPTER 28

CLOTHES TOO TIGHT

What incredible motivation to get out the front door if none of your clothes are fitting like they used to.

First you will be depressed, then you will be shocked, then you will enter the city of hopelessness. I am here to give you a passport out of that city.

Having your clothes become too tight can actually be a blessing for you if it motivates you to do something about it.

Suzanne is a type II diabetic who developed this condition in her late 50s.

She began to put on weight as we tend to do as we grow older. Pretty soon, nothing fit. Pants, dresses, blouses, nothing.

Along with this, her blood sugar was not being controlled well. Extra weight always exacerbates our diabetes.

While she had to purchase new clothes, she also determined to reverse this pattern. She joined Weight Watchers and also began an exercise program that she continues to this day. She lost weight, felt better, and her A1C number fell into the prediabetic range after having been squarely in the diabetic range for years.

And her A1C number stayed there. For years.

All because her clothes became too tight. Listen to your clothes.

CHAPTER 29

EXERCISE THEN REWARD YOURSELF

It might sound silly but rewarding yourself does work on a very basic human principle ...the principle of incentives. Before you laugh, understand that incentives are what our western economy is built on largely. The principle is that incentives bring out the best in human behavior.

So here you are on a Saturday, facing the compelling reasons that you need to exercise to help your diabetes however your inertia has you holed up in your house. Crossing your front door to actually get out and do something seems like mission impossible.

Many people find it very helpful to promise themselves some reward for exercising. It is an incentive. Incentives draw the best out of many of us.

Hey this won't work on me, you say. My friend, give it a try. You are not exempt from the laws of human nature.

Here's an example, you tell yourself that you're going to endure the exercise. You really have zero desire to exercise on that day yet because you're doing it, you promise to reward yourself with something that will motivate you. I can't tell you what that is.

I love books and occasionally I will use the reward of buying a book for my Kindle that I've wanted for a while simply to dangle a carrot in front of me and get me out the front door.

Hey it works and the net here is that I have exercised more by using this technique than by omitting this.

It's all about overcoming the inertia.

CHAPTER 30

THINK OF THE DIABETIC BENEFITS

Early in my career, I was a church worker. As such, I had the benefit of exceptional motivational teachings that I would listen to as various teachers came through my territory.

One teacher stressed the importance of not allowing our feelings to dictate our actions inordinately. He focused on the fact that if we allow our feelings to rule our lives, we would never amount to much of anything or accomplish anything significant.

He stressed that we should operate a great deal out of what we knew as fact that we needed to do as opposed to what we felt. He had a great motto for this… "What you FEEL will make you ill, but what you KNOW will make you go."

Throughout my years, I have always marveled at the wisdom in this saying.

In many ways it applies to motivating us to get out the front door and get exercising.

With that in mind, I think it is vital to reflect on why we are exercising at all. In short, exercising benefits our diabetic condition in so many ways it is impossible to list.

For starters, if you have insulin resistance which most type 2 diabetics do, exercise will lessen that resistance. Exercise will open the receptivity of your cells for blood glucose to enter them. That way it's not in your bloodstream and your blood glucose levels of your blood will fall. That's a good thing.

Diabetes can contribute to a person being depressed. Studies show that walking 20 minutes a day is as therapeutic as most medications or talk therapy. Can you believe that? Well you should because it's true.

Exercise can increase a person's overall fitness level which lessens the comorbidities that can spring up when you deal with diabetes in a person's life.

This alone makes exercise a fabulous, fabulous option for a diabetic.

So think about those mornings when you absolutely do not want to exercise. Your feelings are screaming "do not exercise at all because I do not feel like it". It is mornings like this that what you feel is making you ILL but what you know has got to make you GO. Because you know you need to exercise, you put your feelings up on a shelf and get out the door and get to the business of exercising. Because your intellect is making the smart choice and the smart decision here.

CHAPTER 31

TURN IT FROM A MAYBE TO A MUST ON YOUR CALENDAR

There is something compelling when you schedule something on your calendar. You are more apt to follow through and keep a commitment that is on your calendar than one that is not.

It always helps me to proactively plan my exercise in the future by committing it to my calendar. If you use a paper calendar, pencil it in. If you use an electronic calendar, then schedule it and you will have an automatic reminder.

There is something about human nature that simply makes this work. Let's make it work on our behalf to help us manage our diabetes better.

CHAPTER 32

GET INTO A ROUTINE

One of the most powerful books that I have read regarding the efficacy of habits is called *The Power of Habit* by Charles DuHigg. For those of us who hate exercise, we can harness the power of habitual behavior to move us forward when we do not feel like getting out our front door and exercising.

Once you have found an exercise routine or a group of exercises that work for you, then you can begin building a habit around these. Once you have a habit built around these, it is almost effortless to execute them. And this is what we want, something that is almost effortless. Because that's the type of people we are... we hate exercise or at the very least if we do not hate exercise, we have times of trouble getting motivated to actually do it.

Here is a way to build a habit for those of us that resist such things. Do an exercise or series of exercises for one week daily. Then do it for one more week daily. You now have two weeks of repetitive activity under your belt. Now move into the third week doing the same thing.

You have just launched a new habit.

Some other good books that address the power of habit are:

Discipline Yourself
Mind Hacking
13 Things Mentally Strong People Don't Do

CHAPTER 33

OH NO! RELAPSE!

It all began with an overseas trip to see loved ones.

I was in a great exercise routine, showing up at a local Y every morning quite early and working out of about an hour while my wife did yoga. A great way to start the day!

Until the trip.

When I got back, we just weren't going to the Y in the morning anymore with any regularity.

I had relapsed.

You may find yourself in this predicament also but it is important that you pick yourself up and go back to your routine the very next day. It's hard but it's vital. Inertia cannot win. Inertia cannot win. Inertia cannot win.

You need to throw your perfectionism overboard.

So what if your train runs off the tracks? Of course it will! We are not perfect! Get that train running again!

There's just too much riding on it.

I have a friend who is a very successful dieter. Whenever he falls off the wagon so to speak, he doesn't let it discourage him... rather, he attempts to get back on the wagon as quickly as possible.

It's the same way with exercise. Let's pretend that you are going great for three months and then life hands you a series of events that sidelines you for 3 weeks, where you do no exercise at all. Trust me, this happens.

You are now faced with two options:

1) you can continue doing nothing and all of the incredible benefits that you know will accrue to you will go down the drain.

Or

2) you can get back into your exercise routine.

You need to be flexible with your exercise. Do not make it an all or nothing proposition. If you do not exercise due to circumstances outside of your control, that's okay. Don't let it throw you in the ditch. Be flexible. Get back into your routine as quickly as possible.

You have to end relapse and begin routine again.

You have to take the bull by the horns and remind yourself of the myriad of benefits that exercise is literally raining on you with regards to your diabetes.

Put relapse in the rearview!

You can do it!

CHAPTER 34

VARY EXERCISE

There was a guy that I knew at the local gym who made the following comment to me that sounded profound:

"The way I've been able to keep coming to the gym for 25 years is that I switch it up all the time ... I never do the same exercise 2 days in a row."

Whenever I start initially exercising, one of my most difficult hurdles that I had to face is boredom. It seems like whenever I share this, someone in the group immediately breaks in and says ("that never happens to me!").

So I, like my friend at the gym, have found it to be immensely valuable to vary my exercise in order to keep engaged. What do I mean by that?

Glad you asked, let me tell you.

For example, I may walk briskly for a few days in a row but then I'm a ride my bike for the next week or so. Then I will go back to walking or slow jogging. Then I will grab the barbells and do some strength work.

And then I might swim every other day for the next few days at my local YMCA. And then I made walk again for a couple of weeks every day, always briskly.

Oh I forgot, when I get sick of doing all of that, I might get on the stair step machine at the gym for a few days. What this does is break the routine which always improves motivation.

CHAPTER 35

GET HEADPHONES

Have I mentioned that exercise bores me?

This is one of the reasons why I do not like to exercise... I am one of those people that finds it difficult to engage in anything that is boring. You may not be this type of person however I am.

I find it extremely helpful to be able to distract myself while exercising. I do this by putting on some headphones and either listening to an audiobook, music or a podcast. This lessens my boredom immensely with the added benefit of often learning new things.

And headphones with Bluetooth (hence wireless) are divine.

I have listened to so many audiobooks while exercising that I have lost count.

Why is this motivational? Because it lessens my dread of exercising the next time. If I am able to make my exercise fun, I'm more apt to do it.

CHAPTER 36

YOU TIME

A huge advantage of exercise is that it is an activity that is set aside purely for yourself. You may do it with tons of other people in groups, but you are still doing it for yourself. It is a hugely effective type of "me time".

The great thing about me time is that the more you do it, the more you are motivated to do it. If you begin to look at your exercise as me time, you will be more motivated to engage in it.

Remember, motivation is what we're working on in this book. Overcoming inertia. Getting you off your couch and out the front door.

CHAPTER 37

FIND A PROGRAM TO FOLLOW

I have a friend who says it is in his genetics that whenever he follows a program or any type of structure, his performance improved immeasurably.

I personally find this to be true of myself also. Left to my own devices, often I will drift like a rudderless sailboat in the wind. Add structure to the equation, and my achievement levels skyrocket.

Fitness experts often point to the usage of fitness programs as aids for those of us who need help in being motivated to exercise.

If you are a bit older, the Silver sneakers program is a wonderful walking program to follow.

The couch to 5K program it is a tremendous program for those who want to run but never have done so.

Other programs include:

www.makeyourbodywork.com

www.sweatybetty.com

www.jessicasmithtv.com

www.doyogawithme.com

CHAPTER 38

SAY YOU'LL ONLY WORK OUT FOR 10 MINUTES

I love this one for obvious reasons.

Since I hate all types of exercise and even hate hearing the sound of the word exercise, this really appeals to me. Let me tell you why:

In the business world, there is a process improvement approach called kaizen. In a nutshell, kaizen is built on the philosophy of making improvements through many small steps rather than a few large steps.

Kaizen is very effective in the business world because the smaller the step, the less the pain. However when you add up all the steps together, big change does occur.

There are hundreds of studies that suggest that even working out/exercising in small bursts is hugely beneficial for your diabetic condition. If you cannot walk or exercise for 30 minutes a day to begin, take a 5 minute walk or 10 minute walk. And that's it for the day.

Then do it the next day. Only five or 10 minutes.

Then do it the next day.

A pattern will be established and you will not be put off or intimidated by large parts of the day that you feel you will have to engage in an activity that you don't like.

In other words, starting small is in itself motivational.

Kaizen!

CHAPTER 39

PUT EXERCISE CLOTHES AT FOOT OF BED – MAKE IT EASY

In the business world, especially in those parts where efficiency in movement is crucial, efficiency is often achieved by moving things around to make the movement easier. For example, in a warehouse, the most frequently used items will be stacked the closest to the loading dock in order to save time. And it does save an ENORMOUS amount of time.

There is a principle here that you can leverage in becoming more motivated to exercise…make it easy on yourself.

Here is an example:

Put your exercise clothes at the foot of your bed or somewhere where you can easily reach them. Make it easy to find your exercise clothes. If you are a walker, this might pertain only to your walking shoes. If you are a runner, this would pertain to your running clothes plus your running shoes. If you are doing yoga, this is your mat plus your yoga clothes.

It is all meant to remove a hurdle standing in the way of exercise and make it easier to move into it. Believe it or not, I find this to be motivational in itself… you might not but I do. If I have to run all over the house looking for my clothes, somehow I lose a little bit of motivation and find something else to do.

It is too important for me to exercise to allow this to occur so I see this as a very small step that can yield very large dividends for those of us who hate to exercise.

CHAPTER 40

SELF TALK

There will come that day when you absolutely do not want to begin exercising at all. There are a myriad of reasons that cloud your mind and press you back down to the couch so inertia keeps you from moving out the front door.

These are the tough days that you must tackle and overcome. Your type 2 diabetes may well depend on it. Experience too many of these days and you will lose a valuable ally in your journey to health.

This is when you have to talk to yourself. You have to remind yourself that regardless of how you feel, you must act on what you know. And what you know is that you must get moving.

Oh sure, it is cold outside. And that will make your walk slightly uncomfortable. Or it is raining outside and you must go to your mall or your gym to either walk or workout. But you must overcome this. And you must overcome the inertia by talking to yourself.

Something like this:

I am going to exercise today regardless how I feel.

I really enjoy exercise once I get into it and today will be no different.

I will not let laziness stand in the way of the healthy benefits that I get through exercise

I grow stronger when I exercise, especially when I don't feel like it.

It is amazing how powerful self talk is. It can literally move you from a demotivated sedentary human being to a motivated person getting on with life. And it is all within your power.

CHAPER 41

DRIVE HALFWAY TO THE GYM

I have actually done this on days when inertia and psychological obstacles to exercising seem to be insurmountable.

Here's how it works:

You know you need to go to the gym, you're scheduled to go to the gym, and it is your expectation to go to the gym. But you do not want to go to the gym. And you do not think that there is any way today that you will actually set foot in the gym.

No worries, just jump in your car and drive halfway to the gym. Now turn around and drive back home.

The magic that works for me is that when I am halfway there and about to turn around, I somehow work up the motivation to actually drive the full way there.

Then I usually work out… what I have done is successfully tricked myself however if I did turn around at the halfway point and drive home, at least I had made an effort and that is infinitely better then becoming part of your couch.

CHAPTER 42

ZOO

While writing this book, I had the occasion to go with some family members to the Nashville Zoo one morning.

It was great and I ended up walking at least 3 miles … at least!

I did not notice! I was too caught up in the wonder of this well laid out zoo and all the amazing animals.

I got my exercise in for the day while I did not notice at all! I felt this was too good for me to leave out of this book.

Go to your local zoo and walk through it! You'll be glad you did!

CHAPTER 43

THE QUICK SCIENCE BEHIND IT

WebMD is an excellent resource for diabetics. Here are some quick benefits listed regarding the effect of exercise on diabetes.

- Helps your body use insulin, which controls your blood sugar
- Burns extra body fat
- Strengthens muscles and bones
- Lowers blood pressure
- Cuts LDL ("bad") cholesterol
- Raises HDL ("good") cholesterol
- Improves blood circulation
- Makes heart disease and stroke less likely
- Boosts energy and mood
- Tames stress

When you exercise, your body needs extra energy from blood sugar, also called glucose.

When you do something quickly, like a sprint to catch the bus, your muscles and liver release glucose for fuel.

The big payoff comes when you do moderate exercise for a longer time, like a hike. Your muscles take up much more glucose when you do that. This helps lower your blood sugar levels.

Here is an abstract of a scholarly, peer-reviewed article for those who might like to go a bit deeper into the science behind the magic of exercise on diabetes. (Hint, the last 2 sentences are key)

World J Diabetes. 2014 Oct 15;5(5):659-65. doi: 10.4239/wjd.v5.i5.659.

Acute effects of physical exercise in type 2 diabetes: A review.

Asano RY, Sales MM, Browne RA, Moraes JF,
Coelho Júnior HJ, Moraes MR, Simões HG.

Abstract

The literature has shown the efficiency of exercise in the control of type 2 diabetes (T2D), being suggested as one of the best kinds of non-pharmacological treatments for its population. Thus, the scientific production related to this phenomenon has growing exponentially. However, despite its advances, still there is a lack of studies that have carried out a review on the acute effects of physical exercise on metabolic and hemodynamic markers and possible control mechanisms of these indicators in individuals with T2D, not to mention that in a related way, these themes have been very little studied today. Therefore, the aim of this study was to organize and analyze the current scientific production about the acute effects of physical exercise on metabolic and hemodynamic markers and possible control mechanisms of these indicators in T2D individuals. For such, a research with the following keywords was performed: -exercise; diabetes and post-exercise hypotension; diabetes and excess post-exercise oxygen consumption; diabetes and acute effects in PUBMED, SCIELO and HIGHWIRE databases. From the analyzed studies, it is possible to conclude that, a single exercise session can promote an increase in the bioavailability of nitric oxide and elicit decreases in postexercise blood pressure. Furthermore, the metabolic stress from physical exercise can increase the oxidation of carbohydrate during the exercise and keep it, in high levels, the post exercise consumption of O^2, this phenomenon increases the rate of fat oxidation during recovery periods after exercise, improves glucose tolerance and insulin sensitivity and reduces glycemia between 2-72 h, which seems to be dependent on the exercise intensity and duration of the effort.

CLOSING

I hate to exercise.

I must exercise.

This book has described how I got from point A to point B.

I hope you punch inertia in the face, get off the couch, get into an exercise routine and drop me a line telling me all about it! My email address is terry.blankenship@outlook.com.

For a turbo-charge, follow my blog off-the-couch-today. com. Share with a fellow struggler.

Here's to a wonderful future!

ABOUT THE AUTHOR

Terry Blankenship is a writer/public speaker who lives in Brentwood, TN. A graduate of Owen Graduate School of Management of Vanderbilt University, he has been involved in various aspects of the healthcare industry for over 30 years.

For speaking engagements, contact him at terry. blankenship@outlook.com

Made in United States
Orlando, FL
03 December 2023

40088219R00043